Mastering Canadian Pharmacist Evaluation exam:

Part 1 - Conquering MCQ Evaluation Exams

John Mercola, Bsc Pharm

John Mercola, Bsc Pharm

This book is designed to aid pharmacists aiming to clear the evaluation exam for certification in Canada. It isn't a comprehensive student guide but rather a focused multiple-choice question set tailored to swiftly prepare students for the exams. For those seeking to enhance their understanding in pharmacy and pharmaceutical science, resources like Goodman and Gilman, The Compendium of Pharmaceuticals and Specialties, along with other references, serve as valuable sources. The book assumes that the student is already equipped for the exams and aims to help them test their knowledge while familiarizing them with the types of questions commonly encountered in the exam.

The distribution of questions is as follows:

Biomedical Sciences: 15%

Pharmaceutical Sciences: 25%

Pharmacy Practice: 50%

Behavioural, Social, and Administrative Pharmacy Sciences: 10%

Within these areas, expect questions covering:

Pharmacy Management, which includes Financial, Personnel, Marketing, Quality Improvement, Risk Management, and Workplace Safety

Canadian Healthcare System

Pharmacoeconomics

Biostatistics

This book is crafted as a comprehensive tool to support your journey toward success in the evaluation exams for pharmacist certification in Canada. Its purpose is singular: to bolster your understanding, refine your skills, and fortify your confidence when facing the challenges of these crucial examinations.

However, it's vital to underscore a fundamental principle: this book is not a shortcut to mastery, nor does it supplant the value of your dedication, rigorous study, and hard work. Instead, it's intended as a complementary resource, a guide to augment your preparations and streamline your approach to these exams.

We've meticulously structured this book to align with the examination format, offering a compilation of Multiple Choice Questions (MCQs) tailored to mirror the test's pattern and

complexity. These questions serve as valuable practice exercises, simulating the conditions and scope of the evaluation exams, thereby familiarizing you with the types of queries and enhancing your test-taking skills.

Nevertheless, success in these examinations hinges on more than just familiarity with MCQs. It requires a deep understanding of the diverse facets of biomedical sciences, pharmaceutical sciences, pharmacy practice, behavioural, social, and administrative pharmacy sciences, as well as pharmacy management. Comprehending the Canadian healthcare system, pharmacoeconomics, and biostatistics is equally crucial.

This book's purpose isn't to replace the extensive study required to grasp these subjects. Instead, it serves as a catalyst, allowing you to assess your grasp of the material, identify areas needing further attention, and refine your test-taking strategies.

Remember, your success ultimately hinges on your diligence, perseverance, and commitment to learning. Use this book as a tool in your arsenal, a supplement to your efforts, and a means to gauge your progress.

We encourage you to approach your studies with determination and focus. Engage with the recommended textbooks and references, dive into the intricacies of the subjects, seek guidance when needed, and persist in your pursuit of knowledge.

By combining this book's resources with your unwavering dedication, you'll be better equipped to tackle the evaluation exams and embark confidently on your journey toward becoming a certified pharmacist in Canada.

Wishing you the best in your endeavors.

Warm regards,

John Mercola, Bsc Pharm

Biomedical Sciences

1. Which of the following medications is permitted as a verbal prescription?

a) Hydrocodone

b) Mersyndol (doxylamine, codeine, acetaminophen)

c) Suboxone (buprenorphine/naloxone)

d) Morphine

2. Franklin Brown is a 72 year old male with a complex medication regimen admitted to the hospital for pneumonia. He is taking chlorthalidone, amlodipine, pravastatin and

escitalopram. His blood pressure is 110/70 mm Hg and creatinine clearance is 30 mL/min. The current order is for levofloxacin 750 mg daily every 48 hours x 5 days. Which of the following is NOT one of his QT-prolongation risk factors?

    a) Use of levofloxacin

    b) Use of escitalopram

    c) Use of chlorthalidone

    d) Use of amlodipine

3. Continuing from Question 2, which of the following is an adverse effect of levofloxacin?

    a) Hypertension

    b) Breast tenderness

    c) Tendonitis

    d) Black tongue

4. John Brown received an order for compounded metronidazole suspension for a 22-lb child. The dose is 20 mg/kg/day for 7 days. Using a 5% w/v metronidazole stock solution, how much volume is required for the entire course of the 7 days?

    a) 28 mL

    b) 62 mL

    c) 140 mL

    d) 280 mL

5. Which responsibilities can a pharmacy technician undertake instead of the pharmacist?

a) Receive a verbal prescription for lorazepam

b) Transmit lorazepam to another pharmacy

c) Acquire over-the-counter products from a wholesale supplier

d) Evaluate a patient for potential referral to a walk-in clinic

6. David Myer is a 25 year old male who has trouble sleeping at night due to recent exam stress. Which of the following is suitable advice to assist DN?

a) Napping during the daytime when tired.

b) Reading before bedtime.

c) Exercising during daytime.

d) Drinking alcohol before bedtime.

7. A clinical trial is looking at the incidence of Stevens-Johnson Syndrome among patients given drug X and drug Y. In the drug X group, 10 out of 175 had the adverse effect, compared to 25 out of 170 in the drug Y group. What is the relative risk of developing Stevens-Johnson Syndrome with drug X compared to drug Y?

a) 25%

b) 30%

c) 34%

d) 39%

8. Jerry Roberts is asking for a recommendation for a cough syrup. During the patient interview, it is recommended to avoid confirmation bias with which of the following questions?

a) You are not taking any over-the-counter products currently, right?

b) Do you have any allergies to medications?

c) Is the cough productive or non-productive?

d) What time of the day is the cough most severe?

9. Continuing from Question 8, after interviewing Jerry, you learn he is healthy and on no medications. He developed a phlegm cough 4 weeks ago and started using guaifenesin syrup. His phlegm disappeared within 2 weeks, however, his dry cough remains and keeps him up at night. What is your recommendation for him?

a) Try dextromethorphan instead.

b) Tell him to continue using guaifenesin syrup.

c) Tell him to try behind-the-counter codeine cough syrup.

d) Refer him to a physician for further assessment.

10. Which of the following uses a dangerous abbreviation which the Institute of Safe Medication Practices does NOT approve of?

a) 50 mg

b) 25 µg

c) 0.5 g

d) 15 kg

11. Which of the following is a primary function of the kidneys?

    a. Digestion

    b. Filtration

    c. Respiration

    d. Circulation

12. What is the function of red blood cells?

    a. Oxygen transport

    b. Digestion

    c. Insulin production

    d. Nervous system regulation

13. Which organ is responsible for detoxification of drugs and metabolic waste products?

    a. Heart

    b. Liver

    c. Kidneys

    d. Lungs

14. Which enzyme is responsible for breaking down proteins in the stomach?

    a. Amylase

    b. Lipase

    c. Pepsin

    d. Trypsin

15. What is the basic structural unit of the nervous system?

    a. Neuron

    b. Muscle fiber

    c. Red blood cell

    d. Epithelial cell

16. Which hormone is produced by the thyroid gland and regulates metabolism?

    a. Insulin

    b. Thyroxine

    c. Estrogen

    d. Testosterone

17. What is the primary function of insulin in the human body?

    a. Clotting of blood in human body

    b. Regulation of glucose in human body

    c. Muscle contraction in human body

    d. Bone formation in human body

18. Which of the following is a characteristic of the immune system?

    a. Producing insulin

    b. Fighting infections

    c. Digesting food

d. Regulating body temperature

19. Which vitamin is necessary and imperative for the synthesis of collagen?

a. Vitamin A

b. Vitamin C

c. Vitamin D

d. Vitamin K

20. In human body, what is the role of platelets in the blood?

a. Oxygen transport

b. Clotting

c. pH regulation

d. Immune response

21. Which of the following is a function of the respiratory system?

a. Filtration of blood

b. Oxygen transport

c. Regulation of metabolism

d. Detoxification

22. What is the primary function of the gallbladder?

a. Storage of bile

b. Digestion of proteins

c. Regulation of blood pressure

d. Synthesis of insulin

23. Which hormone is responsible for the fight or flight response?

a. Cortisol

b. Estrogen

c. Melatonin

d. Insulin

24. In human physiology, what is the function of the endocrine system?

a. Regulation of body temperature

b. Communication through hormones

c. Oxygen transport

d. Digestion of carbohydrates

25. Which of the following is an example of a neurotransmitter?

a. Insulin

b. Serotonin

c. Thyroxine

d. Estrogen

26. What is the role of the spleen in the immune system?

a. Production of antibodies

b. Filtration of blood

c. Digestion of fats

d. Storage of glucose

27. What is one of the most important functions of the skeletal system?

a. Oxygen transport

b. Movement and support

c. Digestion of proteins

d. Filtration of blood

28. What is the main function of the thymus gland?

a. Production of insulin

b. Regulation of body temperature

c. Development of T lymphocytes

d. Digestion of fats

29. Which of the following is a component of the central nervous system?

a. Peripheral nerves

b. Spinal cord

c. Skeletal muscles

d. Adrenal glands

30. What is the primary purpose of the lymphatic system?

a. Regulation of blood pressure

b. Filtration of blood

c. Transportation of hormones

d. Immune response

31. Which enzyme is responsible for breaking down carbohydrates in the digestive system?

a. Lipase

b. Amylase

c. Trypsin

d. Pepsin

32. What is the function of the hypothalamus in the brain?

a. Regulation of body temperature

b. Control of hormone secretion

c. Memory storage

d. Muscle coordination

33. Which of the following is considered to be a component of the cardiovascular system?

a. Lungs

b. Liver

c. Pancreas

d. Heart

34. What is the role of the pineal gland?

a. Regulation of blood pressure

b. Production of melatonin

c. Digestion of fats

d. Synthesis of insulin

35. Which of the following is a function of the integumentary system?

a. Oxygen transport

b. Protection against pathogens

c. Filtration of blood

d. Regulation of body temperature

36. What is the primary function of white blood cells in the immune system?

a. Oxygen transport

b. Clotting

c. Fighting infections

d. pH regulation

37. Which of the following is a function of the pancreas?

a. Regulation of body temperature

b. Digestion of proteins

c. Insulin production

d. Filtration of blood

38. What is the role of the parathyroid glands?

a. Production of insulin

b. Regulation of calcium levels

c. Digestion of carbohydrates

d. Synthesis of hormones

39. Which of the following is a component of the peripheral nervous system?

a. Brain

b. Spinal cord

c. Nerves outside the central nervous system

d. Thymus gland

40. What is the function of the corpus callosum in the brain?

a. Regulation of body temperature

b. Coordination of muscle movements

c. Communication between the two hemispheres

d. Digestion of fats

41. Which of the following is a function of the respiratory system?

a. Regulation of body temperature

b. Filtration of blood

c. Oxygen transport

d. Synthesis of hormones

42. What is the role of the adrenal glands in the endocrine system?

a. Production of insulin

b. Regulation of calcium levels

c. Release of stress hormones

d. Digestion of proteins

43. Which of the following is a function of the muscular system?

a. Filtration of blood

b. Oxygen transport

c. Movement of the body

d. Digestion of fats

44. What is the primary function of the cornea in the eye?

a. Regulation of light entering the eye

b. Production of tears

c. Focusing light onto the retina

d. Synthesis of hormones

45. Which organ is responsible for the production of bile?

a. Gallbladder

b. Pancreas

c. Liver

d. Kidneys

46. What is the function of the alveoli in the lungs?

a. Oxygen transport

b. Filtration of blood

c. Gas exchange

d. Synthesis of hormones

47. What role does the excretory system play in the human body in terms of physiological functions?

a. Oxygen transport

b. Filtration of blood

c. Regulation of body temperature

d. Elimination of waste products

48. What is the function of the Eustachian tube in the ear?

a. Regulation of sound waves

b. Equalization of air pressure

c. Production of earwax

d. Synthesis of hormones

49. Which of the following is a function of the pituitary gland?

a. Regulation of body temperature

b. Production of insulin

c. Release of hormones that regulate other glands

d. Digestion of proteins

50. What is the primary function of the mucus in the respiratory system?

a. Oxygen transport

b. Protection against pathogens

c. Digestion of fats

d. Synthesis of hormones

51. Which of the following is a function of the reproductive system?

a. Filtration of blood

b. Oxygen transport

c. Production of gametes

d. Regulation of body temperature

52. What is the primary role of the semicircular canals in the inner ear?

a. Regulation of sound waves

b. Equalization of air pressure

c. Balance and spatial orientation

d. Synthesis of hormones

53. Which of the following is a function of the urinary system?

a. Digestion of proteins

b. Filtration of blood

c. Synthesis of insulin

d. Regulation of body temperature

54. What is the primary function of the lens in the eye?

a. Regulation of light entering the eye

b. Focusing light onto the retina

c. Production of tears

d. Synthesis of hormones

55. Which organ is responsible for the production of insulin?

a. Liver

b. Pancreas

c. Kidneys

d. Thyroid gland

Pharmacy Practice

56. According to Health Canada's interpretation of the legislation and regulations, which of the following activities are pharmacists authorized to conduct with controlled substances under the Controlled Drugs and Substances Act (CDSA)?

a. Adjusting the formulation

b. Prescribing controlled substances

c. Dispensing without a prescription

d. Selling controlled substances without restrictions

57. What does the term "de-prescribing" refer to in the context of pharmacists' activities with controlled substances?

a. Increasing the dosage of a medication

b. The planned and supervised process of reducing or stopping a medication

c. Changing the formulation of a drug

d. Selling medications directly to patients

58. Under the regulations of the CDSA, what is part-filling, as described in the provided information?

a. Disposing of expired medications

b. Refusing to dispense controlled substances

c. Dispensing a quantity less than the total amount specified by a practitioner

d. Providing medications without a prescription

59. According to the provided information, what must pharmacists ensure when conducting activities with controlled substances?

a. Their actions do not restrict patients' access to needed prescriptions

b. Maximizing profits from controlled substance sales

c. Conducting activities without involving prescribing practitioners

d. Selling controlled substances without limitations

60. What is the primary scope of the information provided by Health Canada regarding pharmacists' activities with controlled substances?

a. Legal advice on the Controlled Drugs and Substances Act (CDSA)

b. Guidance to pharmacists and provincial regulators on interpreting the legislation

c. Restrictions on pharmacists' activities with controlled substances

d. Recommendations on maximizing pharmacy profits

61. Which of the following is not available as an over-the-counter (OTC) drug?

A. Salicylates

B. Melatonin

C. Look-alike and act-alike drugs

D. None of the above

62. What is a drug store?

A. A hospital department handling procurement, storage, compounding, and dispensing of drugs and medical devices

B. A hospital department dealing with manufacturing, testing, packaging, and distribution of drugs and medical devices

C. A shop where prescription drugs, over-the-counter medicines, medical devices, and cosmetic and toilet preparations are stored, sold, and dispensed

D. Both a and b

63. What does the Hospital formulary list in a hospital?

A. Instruments

B. Drugs

C. Staff

D. Patients

64. In infants and children, absorption is notably faster than in the neonatal period for which route?

A. Oral

B. Topical

C. Intravenous

D. Intramuscular

65. Which drug does not require therapeutic drug monitoring?

A. Digitoxin

B. Gentamycin

C. Phenytoin

D. Paracetamol

66. The term "Hospital" originated from which Latin word?

A. Asclepieia

B. Hospitale

C. Hospice

D. None of the above

67. How can substantial patient care and financial benefits be increased?

A. Using generic drugs

B. Using branded drugs

C. Both

D. None

68. What is another term for patient care services?

A. Public Health services

B. Allied health services

C. Nursing services

D. Administrative services

69. In a clinical study, who is the sponsor?

A. Country

B. Organization

C. Society

D. Cohort

70. What is the written details for conducting trials to ensure quality control known as?

A. GCP

B. SOP

C. IEC

D. ADR

71. What does the presence of ketone bodies in urine indicate?

A. Kidney dysfunction

B. Nephrosis

C. Hypoglycemia

D. Mushroom poisoning

72. If a 200-bed hospital wants to operate, how many pharmacists should be hired at least?

A. 8

B. 10

C. 15

D. 5

73. What is an appropriate description of Average Costs?

A. The value of opportunities lost by utilizing resources in a particular service or health technology

B. The total costs of a health care system divided by the units of production

C. Independent of the number of units of production and includes heating, lighting, and fixed staffing costs

D. The cost of the consumption of medicines is a good example of variable costs

74. What does Mean Cell Volume represent?

A. Ratio of hematocrit to RBC count

B. Ratio of Hb to RBC

C. Both

D. None

75. Which is an example of a civil hospital?

A. Elite hospital

B. Budget hospital

C. Private hospital

D. Teaching hospital

76. For a 200-bed hospital, how many pharmacists are required?

A. 8

B. 10

C. 15

D. 5

77. Match the following

1. Purchase a. Act of exercise, directing, guiding, or retaining power over

2. Inventory b. Act of obtaining an article by making payments in terms of money

3. Control c. Itemized list of goods with their estimated worth

A. 1-a, 2-b, 3-c

B. 1-b, 2-c, 3-a

C. 1-c, 2-b, 3-a

D. 1-b, 2-a, 3-c

78. According to ICH GCP, how should the investigator be qualified?

A. Training and experience

B. Education, training, and experience

C. Education and experience

D. Education and training

79. What is a pharmaceutical equivalent that produces the same effects in patients?

A. Therapeutic equivalent

B. Therapeutic window

C. Minimum effective concentration (MEC)

D. Minimum toxic concentration (MTC)

80. What is the heart of the patient counseling session?

A. Preparing for the session

B. Opening the session

C. Counseling content

D. Closing the session

81. Which is not a principle of inventory control?

A. Demand Forecasting

B. Accuracy

C. Warehouse flow

D. Overstocking

82. How does the count of hemoglobin change in anemia and leukemia?

A. Increases than normal range

B. Remains constant

C. Decreases than normal range

D. None of the above

83. What are ambulatory patients required to do?

A. Required to admit to the ward for treatment

B. Required to go home after taking treatment in O.P.D.

C. Require emergency treatment

D. None of the above

84. What costs are associated with inventory?

A. Purchase price of the inventory

B. Re-order costs

C. Inventory holding costs, Shortage costs

D. All of the above

85. Which of the following is not an objective of budget preparation?

A. Monitor hospital financial activities

B. Analysis of deviation

C. Development of standards

D. Allowing overexpenditure

86. What is included in the Pharmacy Therapeutic Committee (PTC)?

A. 3 doctors, 1 pharmacist, 1 nursing staff, and hospital administrator

B. 2 doctors, 2 pharmacists, 1 nursing staff, and hospital administrator

C. 2 doctors, 1 pharmacist, 2 nursing staff, and hospital administrator

D. 3 doctors, 2 pharmacists, 2 nursing staff, and hospital administrator

87. What is the duration of long-term and short-term budgets?

A. 2-5 years and 10 years

B. 5 years and 10 years

C. 5-10 years and 2 years

D. 2 years and 5 years

88. Which activity is not included in the role of clinical pharmacists?

A. Attending rounds

B. Studying kinetics of drugs

C. Participating in clinical trials

D. None

89. Which statement is not true about OTC drugs?

A. Are non-prescription drugs

B. Are minimally effective and safe as compared to prescription drugs, which are more potent and frequently dangerous

C. Are easily available

D. None

90. What does DIS stand for?

A. Drug information services

B. Drug implementation services

C. Drug including syndromes

D. Drug incorporation services

91. What is the combination method for codification of various items of drugs?

A. Combination of mnemonic and alphabetical method

B. Combination of mnemonic and numerical method

C. Combination of numerical and letter code method

D. Combination of numerical and alphabetical method

92. What is the average time period for phase II clinical trials study?

A. Up to Four years

B. Up to Few months

C. Up to Two years

D. Up to several years

93. What plays a vital role in drug safety in hospitals?

A. PTC

B. GMP

C. ADR

D. SOP

94. What are the guidelines to achieve drug safety?

A. Dispensing of the medicine

B. Adequate facilities shall be provided for the storage and handling medicine in the pharmacy.

C. All of the above

D. None of the above

95. If you are a pharmacist, which of the following you will not consider as an objective of budget preparation?

A. Monitor hospital financial activities

B. Analysis of deviation

C. Development of standards

D. Allowing overexpenditure

96. What is the objective of Hospital pharmacy?

A. To teach hospital pharmacist about ethics of Hospital Pharmacy

B. To ensure the availability of the right medication at a reasonable cost

C. To attract a greater number of qualified pharmacists to the hospital

D. All of the above

97. Which responsibility of the clinical pharmacist is in the direct patient care area?

A. Supervision of drug administration techniques.

B. Providing drug information to physicians and nurses.

C. Identify drugs brought into the hospital by patients.

D. Reviewing each patient's drug administration forms periodically to ensure all doses have been administered.

98. Which responsibility of the community pharmacist is in the dispensing area?

A. Reviews all doses missed, reschedules the doses as necessary & signs all drugs not given notices.

B. Supervision of drug administration.

C. Ensures that established policies & procedures are followed.

D. Reviewing each patient's drug administration forms periodically to ensure all doses have been administered.

99. The ward pharmacy is controlled by-

A. Satellite Pharmacy

B. Medical officer

C. Nurses

D. Pharmacist

100. Which of the following reactions is called Augmented adverse drug reactions?

A. Genetically determined effects.

B. Idiosyncrasy.

C. Rebound effect on discontinuation

D. Allergic reactions & anaphylaxis.

101. What defines a primary hospital?

A. Less than 100 beds

B. More than 100 beds

C. Less than 50 beds

D. More than 500 beds

102. In a small hospital, what is the minimum number of required pharmacists? A. 4 B. 3 C. 5 D. 6

A. 4

103. For starting a retail drug store, what is the minimum required sq. meter area, and for a wholesale drug store, what is the minimum required sq. meter area? A. 150 and 200

B. 100 and 150 C. 200 and 250 D. None of these

A. 150 and 200

104. What are the various methods employed for codifications? A. Alphabetical order method B. Mnemonic method C. Numerical method D. None of these

C. Numerical method

105. Which drug is contraindicated in pregnancy?

A. Tetracycline

B. Erythromycin

C. Chloroquine

D. Ampicillin

106. What is HBA1c (Glycosylated hemoglobin) a diagnostic test for?

A. Hemoglobin

B. Diabetes mellitus

C. Jaundice

D. Malaria

107. All of the following are cardiac markers except:

A. Ckmb

B. Troponin

C. Myoglobin

D. Bilirubin

108. Which lipoprotein has the highest concentration of cholesterol?

A. VLDL

B. HDL

C. LDL

D. IDL

109. What is the purpose of PTC?

A. Advisory

B. Educational

C. Both A & B

D. Only A

110. Where is a satellite pharmacy located?

A. Each floor

B. For two floors, one pharmacy

C. Only one in a hospital

D. Depends on hospital type

111. What are patients who occupy space in the hospital called?

A. Operating patients

B. Ambulatory patients

C. Inpatients

D. Outpatient

112. Which of the following is not an inventory?

A. Raw material

B. Machine

C. Finished goods

D. Progress goods

113. What is the time period between placing an order and its receipt in stock known as?

A. Lead time

B. Carrying time

C. Shortage time

D. Over time

114. What are the costs associated with inventory?

A. Purchase price of the inventory

B. Re-order costs

C. Inventory holding costs, Shortage costs

D. All of the above

115. What does 'Buffer stock' represent in the level of stock?

A. At which the ordering process should start

B. Half of the actual stock

C. Minimum stock level below which actual stock should not fall

D. Maximum stock in inventory

116. Inventory Control is an important part of which management?

A. Labour

B. Material

C. Expenditure

D. None of the above

117. In ABC analysis, what does the category 'A' include?

A. Weight

B. Value

C. Density

D. Popularity

118. TDM is very essential for those drugs with which kind of therapeutic index?

A. Wide Therapeutic index

B. Large Therapeutic index

C. Narrow Therapeutic index

D. Small Therapeutic index

119. What does clinical pharmacy aim to provide, optimizing the use of medication and promoting health, wellness, and disease prevention?

A. Direct Patient Care

B. Indirect patient care

C. Physician care

D. Product care

120. What does F,S,N stand for in the layout of the drug store?

A. Fast Moving, Slow handling, Non Handling

B. First moving, Second moving, Non moving

C. Fast Storing, Slow Storing , Non storing

D. Fast moving , Slow moving, Non moving

121. What is not a principle of inventory control?

A. Demand Forecasting

B. Accuracy

C. Warehouse flow

D. Overstocking

122. How does the count of hemoglobin change in anaemia and leukemia?

A. Increases than normal range

B. Remains constant

C. Decreases than normal range

D. None of the above

123. What does VED analysis stand for?

A. Very, essential, deal

B. Vital, essential, desirable

C. Very, essential, desirable

D. Vital, essential, deal

124. What does IRB stand for?

A. Institutional Review board

B. International review bureau

C. Indian review board

D. Indian Recognition body

125. What does EOQ stand for?

A. Essential of Quality

B. Economic order quantity

C. Enlist order quality

D. Equipment order quality

126. What are the three critical control levels in inventory control?

A. Reorder level, minimum level and maximum level

B. Reorder level, Safety stock and Average inventory

C. Buffer stock, minimum level and maximum level

D. None of the above

127. What is an increased number of RBC in urine called?

A. Polyuria

B. Oliguria

C. Haematuria

D. Pyuria

128. What is the numerical method also known as?

A. Coding system method

B. Sequence system method

C. Block system

D. Decimal system

129. What is the process of assigning a code number or code symbol to a particular material for easy identification?

A. Decoding

B. Stocking

C. Communicating

D. Coding

130. What type of source is it when information is presented by authors without any evaluation by a second party?

A. Secondary

B. Primary

C. Tertiary

D. Other

131. Why was the Poison Control centre established?

A. To provide rapid access to information valuable in assessing and treating poisonings.

B. Not assist with poisoning prevention.

C. Not manage with the poisoning cases

D. None of the above

132. What quality does a good counselor in patient counseling possess?

A. Be a good listener.

B. Be flexible

C. Be empathetic

D. All of the above

133. What is the benefit of patient counseling?

A. Serving patients and their well-being

B. Improves patient compliance

C. Formation of trusting relationship with patients

D. All of the above

134. What internal teaching program is involved in the training of students in the hospital?

A. Student Nurses

B. Cardiologists

C. Physicians

D. Administrators

135. What is a place where outpatients are provided medical treatment, checkup, or advice for their health?

A. Nursing home

B. Physician home

C. Clinic

D. Hospital

136. In accordance with the regulations governing controlled substances, which healthcare practitioners, possessing specific qualifications and credentials, are granted the authority to prescribe narcotic drugs within the established legal framework?

a. Midwives

b. Chiropractors

c. Osteopaths

d. Pharmacists

137. In a scenario where a pharmacist, holding conscientious objections to emergency contraception, finds themselves solely responsible during a shift when a patient seeks levonorgestrel (Plan B®), what would be the most suitable and ethically responsible course of action for the pharmacist, taking into consideration both their personal beliefs and their professional responsibility to the patient?

a. Recommend a medical assessment at a walk-in clinic before providing the medication.

b. Prioritize the patient's needs, providing the medication on a "once but not again" basis.

c. Prioritize the patient's needs, provide the medication, and set aside personal moral objections.

d. Inform the patient of the inability to provide the medication and direct them to another pharmacy.

138. A pharmaceutical manufacturer offers payment to a pharmacy for hosting a cough and cold information display. What strategy would optimally reduce conflict of interest?

a. Display only the manufacturer's evidence-based products.

b. Ensure session personnel refrain from recommending specific products.

c. Avoid receiving any financial gain for hosting the session on cough and cold products.

d. Have the pharmacist employee supervising the session volunteer without payment.

139. Under federal legislation, which medication requires witnessed destruction in a pharmacy? As per federal law regarding which medicine had been destroyed in a pharmacy setting to abide by regulations and procedures.

a. Ketamine – a powerful anesthetic, which is generally employed both for medical and veterinary reasons, should be correctly managed on disposal with high alertness being necessary on safety due to its regulatory compliance.

b. Duloxetine – A medicine mostly given in dealing with depression and anxiety, should be put and watched by an witness during disposal so as adhere by regulations and avoid people touching it.

c. Galantamine – a drug regularly used in dealing with Alzheimer's disease requires witnessed destruction in the pharmacy to ensure strict regulations are followed and the medicine is not abused or used against any party wrongfully.

d. Toremene – It is a medicine which is for some neuro-medical disorders. Federal laws state how it should be destroyed carefully to avoid falling into wrong hands. So, there should always be witnesses present during disposal because this is why such medicines are controlled.

140. How should the pharmacist document this encounter after KP provides a new prescription for Drug X and identifies a potential interaction? Once the prescriber is consulted, appropriate follow-up measures are determined.

a. No documentation needed if no changes were made to the prescription and the pharmacist deems it appropriate to dispense the medication.

b. Documentation should be avoided to prevent increased liability for the prescriber if an adverse event occurs.

c. Documentation should be made in the patient's pharmacy profile, and the patient should receive a copy of the note to reduce the pharmacist's liability.

d. Comprehensive documentation in the patient's pharmacy profile is imperative, encompassing a detailed account of the monitoring plan for a thorough and organized record-keeping system that aids in patient care and regulatory compliance.

141. According to federal legislation, what is the legally correct refill designation that should be specified on a written prescription for dexamphetamine?

a. Repeat twice

b. Repeat monthly

c. Repeat twice as required

d. Repeat twice at 14-day intervals

142. In accordance with the Benzodiazepine and Other Targeted Substances Regulations, what constitutes the expiration period for renewing a prescription for lorazepam?

a. Six months from the date of prescription issuance

b. Six months from the original dispensing date

c. One year from the date of prescription issuance

d. One year from the original dispensing date

143. What pharmaceutical substance is subject to federal regulation under the Precursor Control Regulations of the Controlled Drugs and Substances Act, recognized as a precursor chemical integral to the production of illicit drugs?

a. Dextromethorphan

b. Dimenhydrinate

c. Diazepam

d. Pseudoephedrine

144. Concerning a drug undergoing research and development processes in Canada, which statement accurately reflects the situation?

a. Application for patent protection is granted for a maximum period of three years.

b. A New Drug Submission must be filed to start clinical trials.

c. Clinical trials involve three phases that assess animal safety and efficacy.

d. Health Canada, under the Food & Drugs Act & Regulations, provides Notice of Compliance.

145. What is the national voluntary organization dedicated to the advocacy of pharmacists and patient care in Canada?

a. Canadian Pharmacists Association

b. Canadian Patient Safety Institute

c. Institute for Safe Medication Practices

d. National Association of Pharmacy Regulatory Authorities

146. According to Health Canada, what comprehensive information should a pharmacist document when administering a vaccine?

a. Date of birth

b. List of other medications

c. Post-immunization adverse effects

d. Drug allergies

147. In the realm of ethical considerations within the pharmaceutical profession, which scenario presents the most significant conflict of interest for a pharmacist?

a. Accepting free training products/devices from a pharmaceutical representative

b. Sharing prescription profits with physicians who recommend the pharmacy to their patients

c. Returning expired products to the manufacturer in exchange for new stock

d. Attending an educational session where refreshments are provided by a pharmaceutical manufacturer

148. In the case of RY, an 85-year-old male residing independently, who seeks guidance regarding the dosage of his diuretic, which closely resembles another tablet, once the pharmacist has provided assistance with his inquiry, what subsequent actions should the pharmacist take to ensure the patient's well-being and safety?

a. Call RY's family doctor to suggest changing the diuretic to something that looks different.

b. Suggest changing the labels on RY's prescription bottles to a bigger font for easier reading.

c. Recommend that the pharmacy use a blister packaging dosette to dispense RY's medications.

d. Suggest that RY write down the answer to his question to avoid future phone calls.

149. In the situation involving JQ, a 67-year-old male effectively managing controlled type 2 diabetes, who records a notably low blood glucose reading of 2.8 mmol/L, and is observed in a confused state by his wife, what specific instructions should JQ's wife be provided to ensure an appropriate response and safeguard the well-being of the patient?

a. Take JQ immediately to the nearest Emergency Department.

b. Have JQ eat a carbohydrate-rich meal and retest in one hour.

c. Give JQ a 15-20 gram glucose supplement and retest in 15 minutes.

d. Retest JQ's blood glucose level in one hour and phone back if it remains low.

150. In the case of RF, an 80-year-old female who develops Clostridioides difficile-associated diarrhea (CDAD) following ciprofloxacin treatment for a urinary tract infection, resulting in severe symptoms, what would be the most suitable therapeutic option for her condition?

a. Oral fidaxomicin

b. Oral metronidazole plus intravenous vancomycin

c. Oral cholestyramine

d. Oral vancomycin plus intravenous metronidazole

151. In the case of CC, a 72-year-old female, who expresses concerns to the pharmacist about recent stomach discomfort while currently on medications including levothyroxine 100 mcg PO daily (for 30 years), acetaminophen 500 mg po qid (for 5 months), atorvastatin 40 mg PO at bedtime (for 4 years), ibuprofen 400 mg po tid prn for joint pain (for 2 months), and zopiclone 3.75 mg po at bedtime prn (for 3 months), which of the following drug therapy problems is most likely contributing to CC's recent symptoms?

a. Too high a dosage of atorvastatin

b. Too high a dosage of zopiclone

c. Use of ibuprofen without gastroprotection

d. Drug interaction between atorvastatin and zopiclone

152. In the case of AM, who has been utilizing bupropion XL 300 mg PO daily for the management of depression without experiencing improvement over the course of four months, and is now advised by the prescriber to transition to citalopram 20 mg po daily, what is the recommended approach for switching antidepressant therapy?

a. Stop bupropion and start citalopram 20 mg daily the next day.

b. Stop bupropion and wait seven days before starting citalopram 20 mg daily.

c. Taper bupropion over seven days and then start citalopram 20 mg daily.

d. Start citalopram 20 mg daily and then taper bupropion dose over seven days.

153. When dispensing a prescription for sumatriptan 100 mg tablets to a patient for the treatment of migraines, what pertinent information should the pharmacist convey to the patient?

a. If sumatriptan does not relieve the headache within four hours, ergotamine may be used.

b. If no relief is achieved in two hours, a dose of 200 mg should be taken.

c. If the headache returns, a dose of 100 mg can be repeated two hours after the first dose.

d. The maximum dosage of sumatriptan 100 mg in any 24-hour period is six tablets.

154. In the situation where JG, who is undergoing chemotherapy, has inadvertently missed her morning dose of metoclopramide 10 mg PO q6h and seeks guidance from the pharmacist, what advice should the pharmacist provide to address the missed dose?

    a. Take the missed dose immediately when she gets home and continue as scheduled.

    b. Take two doses at lunchtime to make up for the missed dose.

c. Skip the missed dose and take the next scheduled dose at lunchtime.

d. Space four doses into the remaining hours between when JG gets home and her bedtime.

155. In the case of EK, a 25-year-old female seeking Plan B® for emergency contraception, what counseling information should the pharmacist offer to ensure comprehensive and informed guidance?

a. Take one tablet daily for three consecutive days.

b. Perform a pregnancy test five days after completing Plan B®.

c. Rely on Plan B® for protection until the next menstrual cycle.

d. Expect spotting a few days after taking Plan B®.

156. Following an interview with a patient at an asthma clinic, what specific findings should be documented in the "plan" section of the SOAP format notes?

a. Nocturnal symptoms

b. Pulmonary test results

c. Dyspnea on exertion

d. Review of inhaler technique at the next visit

157. In the context of evaluating asthma control in a pediatric patient, what multifaceted factors should be taken into account to determine poor control? Specifically, how do the frequency and severity of symptoms, impact on daily activities, presence of nocturnal symptoms, reliance on rescue medications, and the history of exacerbations collectively contribute to the assessment of suboptimal asthma control in children?

a. Number of colds experienced each year

b. Need for use of a spacer device with inhalers

c. Awakening at night with asthma symptoms

d. Keeping one canister of salbutamol at home and one at school

158. What is the primary pathogen frequently associated with acute bacterial rhinosinusitis?

a. E. coli

b. S. aureus

c. S. pneumoniae

d. N. meningitidis

159. In the case of DC, a 57-year-old female prescribed celecoxib 100 mg po bid for osteoarthritis, and currently only taking acetaminophen, while also indulging in wine with dinner, what would be the pharmacist's assessment of DC's newly prescribed therapy?

a. Discontinue acetaminophen with celecoxib use.

b. Discontinue wine consumption with celecoxib use.

c. Require concurrent cytoprotection with celecoxib use.

d. Have no current drug therapy problems.

160.	In the case of BG, a 45-year-old male diagnosed with type 1 diabetes, who employs premixed insulin and notices fluctuating blood glucose values, what would be the most suitable initial adjustment for optimizing BG's insulin regimen?

a. Decrease the suppertime insulin dose.

b. Increase the suppertime insulin dose.

c. Decrease the breakfast time insulin dose.

d. Increase the breakfast time insulin dose.

161.	In the context of a patient undergoing chemotherapy with cisplatin, what represents a significant adverse effect that should be closely monitored?

a. Ototoxicity

b. Hepatotoxicity

c. Photosensitivity

d. Pulmonary fibrosis

162.	Given that cyclosporine inhibits cytochrome P450 isoenzyme 3A4, which medication is susceptible to experiencing elevated serum concentrations when administered concurrently with cyclosporine?

a. Amoxicillin

b. Atorvastatin

c. Metoprolol

d. Levothyroxine

163. In the case of FR, a 70-year-old female experiencing symptoms of nausea, diarrhea, and dizziness after initiating amiodarone, what would be the most suitable recommendation for management and relief of these symptoms?

a. Take loperamide and dimenhydrinate for symptom relief.

b. Increase fluids and bed rest until symptoms resolve.

c. Contact the physician to discontinue amiodarone until symptoms resolve.

d. Contact the physician to suggest a digoxin level test.

164. In the scenario involving FD, a 58-year-old male with hypertension inquiring about the use of cranberry juice for symptoms such as frequent urination, what potential underlying condition could these symptoms suggest, warranting a referral to a physician for further evaluation?

a. Urinary tract infection

b. Prostate hyperplasia

c. Diabetes mellitus

d. Renal complications of hypertension

165. In the case of DS, a 27-year-old male experiencing symptoms of abdominal cramping, fever, and loose stools subsequent to taking clindamycin for a dental abscess, what recommendations should the pharmacist provide to address and manage these adverse effects?

a. These are expected, transient side effects of clindamycin; treat symptoms and continue medications.

b. There may be an interaction between clindamycin and losartan; a pharmacist call to the dentist is warranted.

c. These symptoms may indicate clindamycin-related pseudomembranous colitis; seek immediate medical attention.

d. Symptoms are probably unrelated to DS's medications; treat for flu symptoms and follow up if no improvement.

166. Following the detection of elevated levels of free cortisol in a patient's urine, what constitutes the confirmatory test for establishing the diagnosis of Cushing's syndrome?

a. Budesonide

b. Triamcinolone acetonide

c. Prednisolone

d. Dexamethasone

Pharmacy Management

167. In the case of patients with a history of gastric ulcers requiring daily aspirin (ASA) for stroke prophylaxis, what represents the most effective and appropriate management strategy to address both the need for stroke prevention and the potential risk of gastric ulcers?

a. Concurrent use of an H2 antagonist

b. Use of an enteric-coated product

c. Reduction of the ASA dose to every other day

d. Screening and eradication of H. pylori

168. As per the Pharmacy Act in Canada, which regulatory body possesses the authority to issue, renew, or reinstate a pharmacist's license?

a. Canadian Pharmacists Association

b. National Association of Pharmacy Regulatory Authorities

c. Provincial Regulatory Authority

d. Health Canada

169. In the context of pharmacy ethics, what is the primary responsibility of a pharmacist?

a. Maximizing profits for the pharmacy

b. Ensuring patient confidentiality

c. Promoting patient well-being

d. Advocating for pharmaceutical companies

170. According to the Controlled Drugs and Substances Act, which schedule includes narcotics such as morphine and oxycodone?

a. Schedule I

b. Schedule II

c. Schedule III

d. Schedule IV

171. What is the purpose of the Drug Information Number (DIN) in Canada?

a. Identifying the manufacturer of the drug

b. Uniquely identifying and cataloging drugs approved for sale in Canada

c. Providing information on drug interactions

d. Classifying drugs based on therapeutic categories

172. Under the Food and Drugs Act, which category of drugs requires a prescription for sale to the public?

a. Over-the-Counter (OTC) drugs

b. Controlled substances

c. Prescription drugs

d. Natural health products

173. According to the Benzodiazepine and Other Targeted Substances Regulations, what is the maximum allowable prescription duration for benzodiazepines?

a. One month

b. Three months

c. Six months

d. One year

174. In the context of professional practice, what is the role of a Pharmacy Manager in a pharmacy setting?

a. Dispensing medications only

b. Ensuring compliance with laws and regulations, overseeing staff, and managing workflow

c. Marketing pharmaceutical products

d. Providing clinical consultations to patients

175. According to the National Association of Pharmacy Regulatory Authorities (NAPRA), what is the purpose of the Model Standards for Pharmacy Compounding of Non-Sterile Preparations?

a. Ensuring profitability of compounding services

b. Establishing minimum standards for the compounding of non-sterile preparations

c. Limiting access to compounded medications

d. Promoting collaboration with pharmaceutical manufacturers

176. What information is required on a prescription in Canada to ensure its validity?

a. Patient's phone number

b. Prescriber's signature and license number

c. Pharmacy manager's stamp

d. Drug manufacturer's information

177. According to the Food and Drug Regulations, what is the primary purpose of the Drug Identification Number (DIN) on a drug label?

a. Indicating the expiration date

b. Identifying the drug product and its manufacturer

c. Providing information on potential side effects

d. Classifying the drug based on therapeutic categories

178. In the context of pharmacy management, what does the term "inventory turnover" refer to?

a. The number of times the pharmacy's inventory is sold or used in a given period

b. The process of counting inventory

c. The rate at which new inventory is ordered

d. The total value of the pharmacy's inventory

179. According to the Health Canada regulations, what is the minimum age requirement for the non-prescription sale of acetaminophen in Canada?

a. 12 years

b. 16 years

c. 18 years

d. 21 years

180. Which of the following entities is responsible for accrediting pharmacy technician education programs in Canada?

a. Canadian Pharmacists Association

b. Canadian Council for Accreditation of Pharmacy Programs (CCAPP)

c. National Association of Pharmacy Regulatory Authorities

d. Health Canada

181. What is the primary purpose of the College of Pharmacists in a Canadian province?

a. Marketing pharmaceutical products

b. Ensuring profitability of pharmacies

c. Protecting the public and ensuring the competence of pharmacists

d. Advocating for pharmaceutical companies

182. According to the Food and Drug Regulations, what is the definition of a "new drug" in Canada?

a. Any drug manufactured in the last year

b. A drug that has not been previously sold in Canada

c. A drug that contains a medicinal ingredient not previously approved in Canada

d. A drug with a unique brand name

183. In the context of pharmacy management, what does the term "formulary" refer to?

a. A list of drugs approved for use within a healthcare system or managed care organization

b. The physical layout of the pharmacy

c. The process of drug manufacturing

d. Marketing materials for pharmaceutical products

184. According to the Narcotic Control Regulations, which class of individuals may possess and administer narcotics in the course of their professional practice?

a. Pharmacists only

b. Physicians only

c. Nurse practitioners, midwives, and veterinarians

d. Dentists only

185. What is the primary purpose of the National Association of Pharmacy Regulatory Authorities (NAPRA) in Canada?

a. Ensuring the profitability of pharmacies

b. Harmonizing pharmacy regulations across provinces and territories

c. Marketing pharmaceutical products

d. Providing clinical consultations to patients

186. According to the Personal Information Protection and Electronic Documents Act (PIPEDA), what is a pharmacist's responsibility regarding patient records?

a. Share patient records with pharmaceutical companies for marketing purposes

b. Protect the confidentiality of patient records and obtain patient consent for disclosure

c. Provide patient records to law enforcement without patient consent

d. Use patient records for pharmacy marketing initiatives

187. Which of the following represents a conflict of interest for a pharmacist?

a. Accepting a coffee mug with a pharmaceutical company logo

b. Accepting payment or gifts that may influence professional judgment

c. Attending a pharmaceutical company-sponsored educational event

d. Collaborating with pharmaceutical representatives on patient education materials

188. To whom does the Code of Ethics apply, as stated in the provided information?

a. The Code of Ethics is only applicable to registered pharmacists.

b. The Code of Ethics applies only to pharmacy students and interns.

c. The Code of Ethics applies to all registrants of the College, including registered pharmacists, pharmacy students, interns, and pharmacy technicians.

d. The Code of Ethics is limited to traditional practice settings involving a healthcare professional/patient relationship.

189. Which ethical principle emphasizes the commitment of healthcare professionals to serve and protect the best interests of patients, focusing on the belief that patients seek care with the expectation that professionals will apply their knowledge and skills to improve their well-being?

a. Beneficence (to benefit)

b. Non maleficence (do no harm, and prevent harm from occurring)

c. Respect for Persons/Justice

d. Accountability (Fidelity)

190. What is the focus of the ethical principle of "Beneficence" as outlined in the Ontario College of Pharmacists Code of Ethics?

a. Registrants' commitment to protecting patients from harm

b. Registrants' obligation to actively and positively serve and benefit the patient and society

c. Registrants' respect for patients' autonomy and dignity

d. Registrants' duty to maintain the public trust

191. What does the Principle of Non Maleficence in the Ontario College of Pharmacists Code of Ethics primarily focus on?

a. Registrants' obligation to protect patients and society from harm

b. Registrants' commitment to serving the best interests of patients

c. Registrants' respect for patients' autonomy and dignity

d. Registrants' fiduciary duty to maintain the public trust

192. According to the Code of Ethics, what does the Principle of Non Maleficence require regarding the disclosure of medical errors and "near misses"?

a. Registrants must conceal medical errors to protect their professional reputation.

b. Registrants must disclose medical errors and "near misses" and share information appropriately.

c. Registrants must report medical errors only if they result in significant harm to the patient.

d. Registrants are not responsible for disclosing medical errors.

193. What is the emphasis of the Principle of Respect for Persons/Justice in the Ontario College of Pharmacists Code of Ethics?

a. Registrants' commitment to serving the best interests of patients

b. Registrants' fiduciary duty to maintain the public trust

c. Registrants' dual obligations to respect the intrinsic worth and dignity of every patient and to treat all patients fairly and equitably

d. Registrants' obligation to protect patients and society from harm

194. What does the Principle of Accountability (Fidelity) primarily focus on in the context of the Ontario College of Pharmacists Code of Ethics?

a. Registrants' commitment to protecting patients from harm

b. Registrants' fiduciary duty to be responsible and faithful custodians of the public trust

c. Registrants' respect for patients' autonomy and dignity

d. Registrants' obligation to actively and positively serve and benefit the patient and society

195. Which standard under the Principle of Accountability (Fidelity) emphasizes registrants' responsibility for making reasonable efforts to ensure continuity of patient care?

a. 4.2 Registrants conduct themselves with personal and professional integrity.

b. 4.10 Registrants report professional incompetence or unethical behavior.

c. 4.15 Registrants assume responsibility for making reasonable efforts to ensure continuity of patient care.

d. 4.18 Registrants make fair decisions about the allocation of resources.

196. According to the Code of Ethics, what is the role of registrants in situations where power imbalances exist in professional working relationships?

a. Registrants do not exploit these relationships for personal, physical, emotional, financial, social, or sexual gain.

b. Registrants actively seek to exploit power imbalances for personal gain.

c. Registrants encourage power imbalances to maintain professional authority.

d. Registrants are not responsible for addressing power imbalances.

197. What does the Principle of Accountability (Fidelity) require regarding registrants' participation in public education programs?

a. Registrants are not obligated to participate in public education programs.

b. Registrants participate as appropriate and viable in public education programs that promote health and wellness and disease prevention.

c. Registrants must participate in public education programs, regardless of their relevance.

d. Registrants can only participate in public education programs related to pharmacy practice.

198. What is the primary goal of financial management in a pharmacy setting?

a. Maximizing patient satisfaction

b. Maximizing pharmacy profits

c. Minimizing medication costs

d. Minimizing employee salaries

199. What financial statement provides a snapshot of a pharmacy's financial position at a specific point in time?

a. Income statement

b. Cash flow statement

c. Balance sheet

d. Statement of retained earnings

200. What does the term "inventory turnover" measure in a pharmacy?

a. The speed at which medications are dispensed

b. The frequency of inventory restocking

c. The efficiency of managing pharmacy staff

d. The number of times inventory is sold and replaced within a specific period

201. What is the purpose of a budget in pharmacy management?

a. To control medication prices

b. To allocate resources and control expenses

c. To set pharmacy profit margins

d. To determine employee salaries

202. What is the primary role of a pharmacy manager in personnel management?

a. Maximizing individual employee goals

b. Minimizing staff training

c. Managing and developing pharmacy staff

d. Ignoring employee performance

203. What is the purpose of performance appraisals in personnel management?

a. To determine employee salaries

b. To identify training needs and areas for improvement

c. To eliminate underperforming employees

d. To increase workplace competition

204. What is the primary focus of workforce diversity in pharmacy management?

a. Minimizing differences among employees

b. Promoting a homogenous work environment

c. Recognizing and valuing differences among employees

d. Ignoring cultural factors in the workplace

Answer: c. Recognizing and valuing differences among employees

205. What does the term "workplace culture" refer to in pharmacy management?

a. The physical layout of the pharmacy

b. The values, beliefs, and behaviors of employees

c. The number of employees in the pharmacy

d. The types of medications dispensed

206. In the context of pharmacy marketing, what is the purpose of market

segmentation?

a. To decrease competition

b. To target specific customer groups with tailored marketing strategies

c. To reduce the variety of products offered

d. To limit the geographic reach of the pharmacy

207. What is the role of social media in pharmacy marketing?

a. Increasing medication prices

b. Minimizing customer engagement

c. Enhancing communication with customers and promoting services

d. Restricting customer access to information

208. What does the term "SWOT analysis" stand for in pharmacy marketing?

a. Strengths, Weaknesses, Opportunities, Threats

b. Sales, Workforce, Operations, Technology

c. Strategies, Wins, Objectives, Trends

d. Scheduling, Workload, Organization, Training

209. How does a loyalty program contribute to pharmacy marketing?

a. By discouraging customer loyalty

b. By offering discounts and rewards to frequent customers

c. By limiting customer access to products

d. By increasing medication prices

210. What is the primary goal of a continuous quality improvement (CQI) program in

pharmacy practice?

a. Maximizing individual employee goals

b. Identifying and rectifying problems in pharmacy processes

c. Ignoring customer feedback

d. Minimizing medication dispensing

211. What does the acronym DMAIC stand for in the context of quality improvement?

a. Define, Measure, Analyze, Improve, Control

b. Data, Management, Analysis, Integration, Collaboration

c. Design, Monitor, Assess, Implement, Control

d. Document, Measure, Analyze, Implement, Correct

212. What role does benchmarking play in quality improvement in pharmacy management?

a. Setting unrealistic goals for the pharmacy

b. Comparing pharmacy performance against industry standards or best practices

c. Ignoring customer feedback

d. Limiting employee involvement in quality improvement

213. What is the primary purpose of root cause analysis in quality improvement?

a. Blaming individual employees for errors

b. Identifying the underlying causes of problems or errors

c. Avoiding responsibility for pharmacy mistakes

d. Disregarding customer complaints

214. What is the purpose of a risk management plan in pharmacy practice?

a. Maximizing patient satisfaction

b. Identifying and minimizing potential risks to patients and the pharmacy

c. Ignoring potential legal issues

d. Reducing employee salaries

215. What does the term "medication error" refer to in the context of risk management?

a. A deliberate act to harm a patient

b. Any preventable event that may cause or lead to inappropriate medication use or patient harm

c. A routine practice in pharmacy

d. The intentional mislabeling of medications

216. How does the use of barcoding technology contribute to risk management in pharmacy practice?

a. Increases the risk of medication errors

b. Reduces the need for prescription verification

c. Enhances medication safety by reducing errors in medication dispensing

d. Limits the types of medications dispensed

217. What is the role of incident reporting in risk management?

a. Discouraging employees from reporting errors

b. Identifying and addressing potential risks and errors

c. Punishing employees for mistakes

d. Minimizing patient involvement in risk management

218. What is the primary goal of occupational health and safety programs in pharmacy practice?

a. Maximizing patient satisfaction

b. Providing a safe and healthy work environment for employees

c. Ignoring workplace hazards

d. Reducing employee salaries

219. What is the purpose of personal protective equipment (PPE) in pharmacy practice?

a. Maximizing patient satisfaction

b. Enhancing employee comfort

c. Providing a barrier against workplace hazards

d. Limiting employee access to medications

220. How does a safety data sheet (SDS) contribute to workplace safety in a pharmacy?

a. By providing information on employee salaries

b. By detailing the hazardous properties of substances in the workplace

c. By minimizing employee involvement in safety measures

d. By reducing the number of safety protocols

221. What is the primary purpose of fire safety training in pharmacy practice?

a. Maximizing patient satisfaction

b. Reducing employee salaries

c. Providing employees with the knowledge and skills to respond to a fire emergency

d. Ignoring workplace hazards

222. What is the purpose of a break-even analysis in pharmacy financial management?

a. Maximizing patient satisfaction

b. Identifying the point at which total revenue equals total costs

c. Reducing employee salaries

d. Minimizing medication prices

223. What is the primary goal of a mentoring program in pharmacy personnel

management?

a. Minimizing employee training costs

b. Providing a structured way for experienced employees to guide and support less experienced

employees

c. Ignoring the professional development of employees

d. Reducing employee salaries

224. How does community involvement contribute to pharmacy marketing?

a. By discouraging customer engagement

b. By increasing medication prices

c. By building positive relationships with the community and attracting customers

d. By limiting access to pharmacy services

225. What is the primary purpose of a root cause analysis in quality improvement?

a. Blaming individual employees for errors

b. Identifying the underlying causes of problems or errors

c. Avoiding responsibility for pharmacy mistakes

d. Disregarding customer complaints

226. How does the implementation of technology contribute to risk management in pharmacy practice?

a. By increasing the risk of medication errors

b. By reducing the need for employee training

c. By enhancing medication safety and minimizing errors

d. By limiting access to pharmacy information

227. What is the purpose of an emergency evacuation plan in pharmacy workplace safety?

a. Minimizing patient satisfaction

b. Reducing employee salaries

c. Providing guidelines for employees to exit the workplace safely in case of an emergency

d. Ignoring workplace hazards

228. What role does hazard communication training play in workplace safety?

a. Increasing the risk of workplace accidents

b. Reducing the need for safety protocols

c. Ensuring that employees understand the hazards associated with the substances they work with

d. Ignoring employee safety concerns

229. How does a safety committee contribute to workplace safety in a pharmacy?

a. By discouraging employee involvement in safety measures

b. By eliminating the need for safety protocols

c. By providing a forum for employees to discuss and address safety concerns

d. By increasing workplace hazards

What is the purpose of regular safety inspections in pharmacy workplace safety?

a. Minimizing patient satisfaction

b. Reducing employee salaries

c. Identifying and addressing potential safety hazards in the workplace

d. Ignoring workplace safety regulations

230. How does a culture of safety contribute to workplace safety in pharmacy practice?

a. By promoting a disregard for safety protocols

b. By minimizing the importance of employee safety

c. By fostering an environment where employees prioritize safety and report concerns

d. By increasing workplace accidents

Pharmaceutical Sciences

231. Which of the following is NOT a type of dosage form?

a. Tablet

b. Elixir

c. Transduction

d. Ointment

232. What is the primary role of excipients in pharmaceutical formulations?

a. Provide color to the formulation

b. Improve taste of the drug

c. Contribute to the therapeutic effect

d. Aid in the formulation and stability of the drug product

233. Which class of drugs inhibits the activity of angiotensin-converting enzyme (ACE)?

a. Beta blockers

b. Diuretics

c. ACE inhibitors

d. Calcium channel blockers

234. The process of converting a drug from its salt form to a free base is known as:

a. Salting out

b. Salt formation

c. Salt disproportionation

d. Saline conversion

235. What is the purpose of the Pharmacists' Gateway Canada?

a. To provide continuing education for pharmacists

b. To facilitate the registration process for internationally educated pharmacists

c. To regulate the pharmaceutical industry in Canada

d. To promote over-the-counter medications

236. Which of the following is an example of a Schedule II controlled substance in Canada?

a. Acetaminophen

b. Codeine

c. Ibuprofen

d. Aspirin

237. What is the primary function of the liver in drug metabolism?

a. Excretion of drugs

b. Activation of prodrugs

c. Inactivation of drugs

d. Absorption of drugs

238. Which regulatory body in Canada is responsible for approving new drugs?

a. Health Canada

b. Canadian Pharmacists Association

c. Canadian Institutes of Health Research

d. Canadian Medical Association

239. What is the therapeutic index of a drug?

a. The ratio of the drug's toxic dose to its therapeutic dose

b. The ratio of the drug's therapeutic dose to its maximum tolerated dose

c. The ratio of the drug's efficacy to its safety

d. The ratio of the drug's half-life to its duration of action

240. Which vitamin is synthesized in the skin upon exposure to sunlight?

a. Vitamin A

b. Vitamin C

c. Vitamin D

d. Vitamin E

241. What is the primary mechanism of action of statin medications?

a. Inhibition of cholesterol synthesis

b. Enhancement of insulin sensitivity

c. Inhibition of blood clotting

d. Relaxation of smooth muscle

242. Which phase of clinical trials involves a small group of healthy volunteers and focuses on dosage range finding?

a. Phase I

b. Phase II

c. Phase III

d. Phase IV

243. What is the purpose of the National Drug Scheduling Advisory Committee (NDSAC)?

a. To regulate the import and export of pharmaceuticals

b. To assess the therapeutic efficacy of new drugs

c. To recommend the scheduling of drugs under the Controlled Drugs and Substances Act

d. To conduct post-market surveillance of pharmaceutical products

244. Which of the following is a common side effect of nonsteroidal anti-inflammatory drugs (NSAIDs)?

a. Constipation

b. Hypertension

c. Photosensitivity

d. Dry mouth

245. In pharmaceutical compounding, what does the term "levigation" refer to?

a. Mixing a drug with a small amount of liquid to form a smooth paste

b. Reducing the particle size of a drug by grinding it with a mortar and pestle

c. Dissolving a drug in a suitable solvent

d. Creating a stable emulsion of oil and water

246. Which of the following is a second-generation antipsychotic medication?

a. Haloperidol

b. Risperidone

c. Amitriptyline

d. Lorazepam

247. What is the primary function of the Canadian Society of Hospital Pharmacists (CSHP)?

a. Accreditation of pharmacy schools

b. Promotion of research in pharmaceutical sciences

c. Advancement of hospital pharmacy practice

d. Regulation of pharmacy technicians

248. Which of the following statements about drug interactions is true?

a. Drug interactions always result in increased therapeutic effects.

b. Drug interactions are only relevant for prescription medications.

c. Drug interactions can lead to increased or decreased therapeutic effects or adverse effects.

d. Drug interactions only occur at high doses of medications.

249. What is the primary role of the Pan-Canadian Pharmaceutical Alliance (pCPA)?

a. To regulate the pricing of pharmaceuticals in Canada

b. To negotiate joint procurement agreements for brand-name and generic drugs

c. To conduct post-marketing surveillance of pharmaceutical products

d. To accredit pharmacy schools in Canada

250. Question: Which of the following is an example of a biologic drug?

a. Atorvastatin

b. Insulin glargine

c. Metformin

d. Warfarin

251. What is the primary function of P-glycoprotein in drug metabolism?

a. Drug absorption

b. Drug excretion

c. Drug metabolism

d. Drug distribution

252. Which class of antibiotics inhibits bacterial cell wall synthesis?

a. Tetracyclines

b. Macrolides

c. Penicillins

d. Fluoroquinolones

253. What is the main purpose of a stability study in pharmaceutical development?

a. To assess the pharmacokinetics of a drug

b. To evaluate the safety profile of a drug

c. To determine the shelf life of a drug product

d. To investigate the drug's mechanism of action

254. Which dosage form is designed to release its active ingredient in a controlled manner over an extended period?

a. Immediate-release tablet

b. Enteric-coated capsule

c. Sustained-release tablet

d. Effervescent granules

255. What is the primary mechanism of action of anticoagulant medications?

a. Inhibition of platelet aggregation

b. Inhibition of blood clotting factors

c. Enhancement of fibrinolysis

d. Vasoconstriction

256. Which vitamin is essential for the synthesis of collagen and wound healing?

a. Vitamin A

b. Vitamin C

c. Vitamin D

d. Vitamin K

257. Which regulatory body oversees the practice of pharmacy in Canada?

a. Health Canada

b. Canadian Pharmacists Association

c. National Association of Pharmacy Regulatory Authorities (NAPRA)

d. Canadian Institutes of Health Research

258. What is the primary role of the Canadian Agency for Drugs and Technologies in Health (CADTH)?

a. Drug approval

b. Drug pricing

c. Health technology assessment

d. Post-market surveillance

259. Which of the following is a common side effect of angiotensin-converting enzyme (ACE) inhibitors?

a. Hyperkalemia

b. Hypoglycemia

c. Hypercalcemia

d. Hypertension

260. What is the purpose of the Drug Identification Number (DIN) in Canada?

a. To identify the manufacturer of a drug

b. To track the distribution of a drug

c. To indicate the therapeutic class of a drug

d. To allow the sale of a drug in Canada

261. Which of the following is an example of a biopharmaceutical dosage form?

a. Sublingual tablet

b. Metered-dose inhaler

c. Buccal patch

d. Intravenous infusion

262. In pharmaceutical compounding, what is the purpose of a surfactant?

a. Increase drug solubility

b. Enhance drug stability

c. Decrease drug absorption

d. Improve drug taste

263. Which of the following is an example of a specialty pharmacy service?

a. Community pharmacy

b. Hospital pharmacy

c. Compounding pharmacy

d. Mail-order pharmacy

264. What is the role of the Patented Medicine Prices Review Board (PMPRB) in

Canada?

a. To approve new drug formulations

b. To regulate the prices of patented medicines

c. To conduct clinical trials for new drugs

d. To provide post-marketing surveillance

265. Which of the following is a common adverse effect associated with opioids?

a. Hypertension

b. Hypoglycemia

c. Respiratory depression

d. Gastrointestinal bleeding

266. What is the primary purpose of the Canadian Council for Accreditation of Pharmacy Programs (CCAPP)?

a. To regulate the practice of pharmacy

b. To accredit pharmacy schools

c. To conduct research in pharmaceutical sciences

d. To provide continuing education for pharmacists

267. Which of the following is a common side effect of proton pump inhibitors (PPIs)?

a. Diarrhea

b. Constipation

c. Osteoporosis

d. Tachycardia

268. What is the primary function of the Canadian Society of Pharmacology and Therapeutics (CSPT)?

a. Regulation of drug pricing

b. Promotion of pharmacology research

c. Accreditation of pharmacy technicians

d. Assessment of drug safety

269. Which phase of clinical trials involves a large number of patients to assess the drug's effectiveness, safety, and side effects?

a. Phase I

b. Phase II

c. Phase III

d. Phase IV

270. What is the primary purpose of Good Manufacturing Practice (GMP) in the pharmaceutical industry?

a. Ensuring the safety and efficacy of drug products

b. Controlling drug pricing

c. Regulating drug advertising

d. Facilitating drug import and export

Behavioural, Social and Administrative Pharmacy Sciences

271. What is the primary focus of Behavioral Pharmacy?

a. Drug development

b. Patient behavior and medication use

c. Pharmaceutical care

d. Drug interactions

272. In the Health Belief Model, what factor influences an individual's decision to take action to prevent or control illness?

a. Perceived susceptibility

b. Perceived benefits

c. Perceived barriers

d. Self-efficacy

273. Which of the following is an example of a cognitive-behavioral strategy to improve medication adherence?

a. Providing medication reminders

b. Offering financial incentives

c. Using motivational interviewing techniques

d. Dispensing medications in blister packs

274. The Theory of Planned Behavior includes which of the following as a key determinant of behavior?

a. Attitude

b. Self-efficacy

c. Perceived control

d. Social norms

275. Which branch of pharmacy focuses on the social aspects of pharmaceutical care, including patient counseling and education?

a. Social Pharmacy

b. Community Pharmacy

c. Clinical Pharmacy

d. Administrative Pharmacy

276. What is the primary goal of medication therapy management (MTM) services?

a. Maximizing pharmacy profits

b. Improving patient outcomes through optimized medication use

c. Reducing medication access

d. Minimizing patient involvement in treatment decisions

277. In the Transtheoretical Model of Change, which stage involves maintaining a behavior change over time?

a. Precontemplation

b. Contemplation

c. Action

d. Maintenance

278. What is the primary purpose of formulary management in pharmacy practice?

a. Maximizing pharmaceutical industry profits

b. Controlling medication costs and ensuring their availability

c. Limiting patient access to medications

d. Expanding the range of available medications

279. Which of the following is a key principle of patient-centered care in pharmacy practice?

a. Minimizing patient involvement in decision-making

b. Focusing solely on disease-oriented outcomes

c. Considering patient preferences and values

d. Ignoring cultural and social factors

280. What is the role of a pharmacy benefit manager (PBM) in the healthcare system?

a. Direct patient care

b. Medication manufacturing

c. Medication pricing and reimbursement

d. Pharmacy education

281. Which of the following is a component of the Systems Theory in healthcare?

a. Focus on individual components in isolation

b. Emphasis on linear cause-and-effect relationships

c. Recognition of the interdependence of components within a system

d. Minimization of feedback loops

282. What does the acronym PDSA stand for in the context of quality improvement in healthcare?

a. Plan-Do-Study-Act

b. Patient-Doctor-System-Analysis

c. Pharmacy-Dispensing-Storage-Audit

d. Prevention-Diagnosis-Symptom-Analysis

283. In the context of patient safety, what does the term "medication reconciliation" refer to?

a. Verifying the accuracy of patient insurance information

b. Ensuring that patients are aware of potential side effects of medications

c. Comparing a patient's medication orders to all the medications that the patient has been taking

d. Assessing patient adherence to prescribed medications

284. What is the primary purpose of a pharmacy and therapeutics (P&T) committee?

a. Maximizing pharmacy profits

b. Evaluating and selecting medications for formulary inclusion

c. Providing direct patient care

d. Conducting medication research

285.   Which of the following is a component of cultural competence in healthcare?

a. Ignoring cultural differences to maintain objectivity

b. Recognizing and respecting cultural differences

c. Promoting a one-size-fits-all approach to patient care

d. Assuming that all patients from a particular cultural group have the same beliefs and values

286.   What is the primary purpose of a medication therapy review (MTR) in pharmacy practice?

a. Maximizing pharmacy profits

b. Identifying drug interactions and adverse effects

c. Promoting medication non-adherence

d. Reducing patient involvement in treatment decisions

287.   In the context of healthcare policy, what does the acronym HIPAA stand for?

a. Health Information Protection and Accountability Act

b. Healthcare Information Privacy and Accessibility Act

c. Health Insurance Portability and Accountability Act

d. Healthcare Insurance Protection and Accessibility Act

288. What is the primary goal of a medication synchronization program in community pharmacy?

a. Maximizing pharmacy profits

b. Improving medication adherence by aligning refill dates

c. Limiting patient access to medications

d. Reducing the range of available medications

289. In the context of healthcare communication, what does the acronym SBAR stand for?

a. Situation, Background, Assessment, Recommendation

b. Systematic, Brief, Analysis, Response

c. Structure, Background, Analysis, Response

d. Support, Briefing, Assessment, Response

290. Which of the following is a component of the Community Reinforcement Approach and Family Training (CRAFT) model for substance abuse treatment?

a. Enabling behavior

b. Punishment and confrontation

c. Positive reinforcement for non-substance use

d. Isolation and withdrawal

291. In the context of pharmacy practice, what does the term "pharmaceutical care" refer to?

a. Maximizing pharmacy profits

b. Focusing solely on dispensing medications

c. Patient-centered practice aimed at optimizing medication use and improving health outcomes

d. Limiting patient access to medications

292. What is the primary focus of health economics in pharmacy practice?

a. Maximizing pharmacy profits

b. Assessing the cost-effectiveness of healthcare interventions

c. Promoting high-cost medications

d. Reducing patient access to medications

293. Which of the following is a key concept in the Social Cognitive Theory of behavior change?

a. Self-determination

b. Reciprocal determinism

c. Learned helplessness

d. Psychoanalytic theory

294. What is the primary purpose of a medication access program in pharmacy practice?

a. Maximizing pharmacy profits

b. Providing free medications to patients

c. Limiting patient access to medications

d. Promoting medication non-adherence

295. In the context of healthcare disparities, what does the term "cultural competence" refer to?

a. Ignoring cultural differences to maintain objectivity

b. Recognizing and respecting cultural differences in patient care

c. Promoting a one-size-fits-all approach to patient care

d. Assuming that all patients from a particular cultural group have the same beliefs and values

296. What is the primary goal of medication therapy adherence clinics in pharmacy practice?

a. Maximizing pharmacy profits

b. Assessing patient adherence to prescribed medications

c. Promoting medication non-adherence

d. Limiting patient access to medications

297. Which of the following is a component of the Health Literacy Universal Precautions Toolkit?

a. Simplify communication

b. Use medical jargon

c. Provide complex written materials

d. Disregard patient preferences

298. In the context of healthcare policy, what does the acronym CMS stand for?

a. Center for Medicare and Social Services

b. Canadian Medical System

c. Centers for Medicare & Medicaid Services

d. Community Medical Standards

299. What is the primary purpose of a medication therapy management (MTM) program in pharmacy practice?

a. Maximizing pharmacy profits

b. Assessing patient adherence to prescribed medications

c. Optimizing medication therapy to improve patient outcomes

d. Limiting patient access to medications

300. Question: Which of the following is a key concept in the Theory of Reasoned Action?

a. Perceived susceptibility

b. Subjective norm

c. Self-efficacy

d. Perceived control

Answers

1. B	2. D	3. C	4. D	5. D	6. C	7. D	8. C	9.A	10. B	11. B	12. A
13. B	14. C	15. A	16. B	17. B	18. B	19. C	20. B	21. B	22. A	23. A	24. B
25. B	26. A	27. B	28. C	29. B	30. C	31. A	32. A	33. D	34. B	35. B	36. C
37. C	38. A	39. C	40. B	41. C	42. C	43. C	44. C	45. C	46 .C	47. D	48. B
49. C	50. B	51. C	52. C	53. B	54. B	55. B	56. A	57. B	58. C	59. A	60. B
61. D	62. C	63. B	64. A	65. D	66. B	67. A	68. C	69. B	70. B	71. C	72. 8
73. B	74. A	75. D	76. A	77. B	78. B	79. A	80. C	81. B	82. C	83. B	84. D
85. D	86. A	87. C	88. D	89. B	90. A	91. B	92. C	93. A	94. C	95. D	96. D
97. D	98. B	99. C	100. C	101. B	102. A	103. A	104. C	105. A	106. B	107. D	108. C
109. C	110. A	111. C	112. B	113. A	114. D	115. C	116. B	117. B	118. C	119. A	120. B
121.D	122. C	123. B	124. A	125. B	126. B	127. C	128. D	129. D	130. B	131. A	132. D
133.D	134. A	135. C	136. A	137. D	138. C	139. A	140. D	141. D	142. C	143. D	144. D
145. A	146. C	147. B	148. C	149. C	150. A	151. C	152. C	153. C	154. C	155. D	156. D
157. C	158. C	159. D	160. A	161.A	162. B	163. D	164. C	165. C	166. D	167. D	168. C
169. C	170. C	171. B	172. C	173. B	174. B	175. B	176. B	177. B	178. A	179. C	180. B
181. C	182. C	183. A	184. C	185. B	186. B	187. B	188. C	189. A	190. B	191. A	192. B
193. C	194. B	195. C	196. A	197. B	198. B	199. B	200. D	201. B	202. C	203. B	204. C
205. B	206. B	207. C	208. A	209. B	210. B	211. A	212. B	213. B	214. B	215. B	216. C
217. B	218. B	219. C	220. B	221. C	222. B	223. B	224. C	225. B	226. C	227. C	228. C

229. C	230. C	231. C	232. D	233. C	234. A	235. B	236. B	237. C	238. A	239. A	240. C
241. A	242. A	243. C	244. B	245. B	246. B	247. C	248. C	249. B	250. B	251. B	252. C
253. C	254. C	255. B	256. B	257. C	258. C	259. A	260. D	261. B	262. A	263. D	264. B
265. C	266. B	267. C	268. B	269. C	270. A	271. B	272. C	273. C	274. C	275. A	276. B
277. D	278. B	279. C	280. C	281. C	282. A	283. C	284. B	285. B	286. B	287. C	288. B
289. A	290. C	291. C	292. B	293. B	294. B	295. B	296. B	297. A	298. C	299. C	300. B